# THE MOST EXTREME ACID REFLUX COOKBOOK FOR SENIORS

Easy Delicious and Healthy Recipe guide, Meal plan with Comprehensive Strategies to Effectively be eased from GERD and  LPR…

**BY**

**Mildred Kent**

**TABLE OF CONTENT**

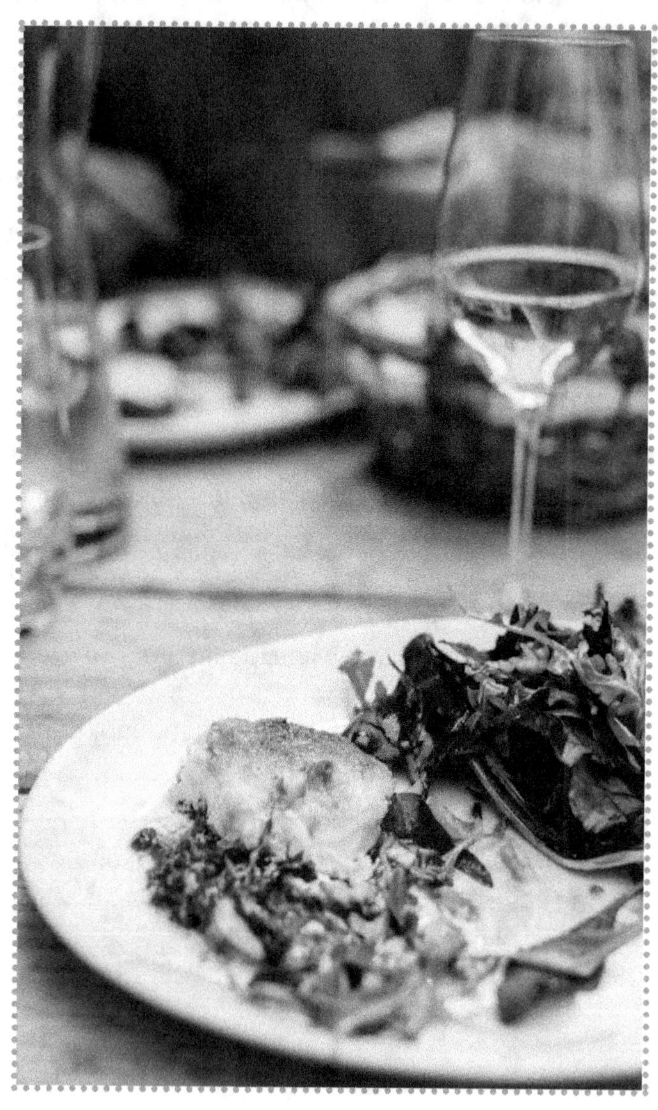

# CHAPTER ONE

## 1. Introduction to Acid Reflux

Stomach acid flowing back into the esophagus is a common digestive disorder known as acid reflux, also known as gastroesophageal reflux disease (GERD). This backflow of acid can cause irritation and inflammation of the esophageal lining, leading to various symptoms such as heartburn, regurgitation, and chest pain.

### 1.1 Understanding Acid Reflux: Causes and Symptoms

The emergence of acid reflux can be attributed to multiple factors. One primary cause is a weakening of the lower esophageal sphincter (LES), a muscular valve that normally prevents stomach acid from flowing back into the esophagus. When the LES becomes relaxed or weakened, it allows stomach acid to reflux into the esophagus, resulting in symptoms.

Other factors that can trigger or exacerbate acid reflux include:

1. **Dietary Choices:** Certain foods and beverages, such as spicy foods, citrus fruits, caffeine, alcohol, and fatty or fried foods, can relax

the LES or stimulate excess acid production, making reflux more likely.

2. **Lifestyle Habits:** Smoking, obesity, and lying down immediately after eating can increase pressure on the stomach, promoting acid reflux.

3. **Medical Conditions:** Hiatal hernia, pregnancy, and certain medical conditions like scleroderma or gastroparesis can also contribute to the development of acid reflux.

Although they can differ from person to person, acid reflux symptoms frequently include:

- **Heartburn:** A burning feeling in the chest that could get worse while you're sleeping or eating.

-**Regurgitation:** The feeling of acid refluxing back into the mouth or throat.

- **Dysphagia:** Difficulty swallowing.

- **Chest Pain:** Sharp or burning pain in the chest, often mistaken for a heart attack.

- **Chronic Cough:** A persistent cough that may be worsened by lying down or eating.
- **Hoarseness:** Changes in the voice due to irritation of the vocal cords by stomach acid.

## 1.2    Impact of Acid Reflux on Digestive Health

Untreated acid reflux can have significant consequences for digestive health. The chronic exposure of the esophagus to stomach acid can lead to complications such as:

1. **Esophagitis:** Inflammation and irritation of the esophageal lining, which can cause pain and difficulty swallowing.

2. **Esophageal Strictures:** Narrowing of the esophagus due to scarring from repeated acid exposure, making swallowing difficult.

3. **Barrett's Esophagus:** A condition in which the cells lining the lower esophagus change in response to acid exposure, increasing the risk of esophageal cancer.

4. **Respiratory Problems:** Aspiration of stomach acid into the lungs can lead to respiratory issues such as asthma, pneumonia, or chronic cough.

Moreover, the symptoms of acid reflux can significantly impact quality of life, leading to sleep disturbances, reduced productivity, and decreased overall well-being.

## 1.3   Importance of Diet in Managing Acid Reflux

One of the key strategies for managing acid reflux is adopting a healthy diet that minimizes reflux triggers and promotes digestive health. Here are some dietary guidelines to help manage acid reflux:

1. **Avoid Trigger Foods:** Identify and avoid foods and beverages that trigger your acid reflux symptoms. Common triggers include spicy foods, citrus fruits, tomatoes, coffee, alcohol, chocolate, and fatty or fried foods.

2. **Eat Smaller Meals:** Consuming smaller, more frequent meals can help prevent excessive stomach distension and reduce the likelihood of acid reflux.

3. **Limit Acidic Foods:** Limit your intake of acidic foods and beverages, such as citrus fruits, tomatoes, and vinegar, as they can exacerbate acid reflux symptoms.

4. **Choose Low-Fat Options:** Opt for lean proteins and low-fat dairy products, as fatty foods can delay stomach emptying and increase the risk of reflux.

5. **Stay Hydrated:** Drink plenty of water throughout the day to help dilute stomach acid and promote healthy digestion.

6. **Eat Mindfully:** Take your time when eating, and chew your food thoroughly. Avoid eating large meals before bedtime, as lying down can exacerbate reflux symptoms.

7. **Consider Dietary Supplements:** Some supplements, such as melatonin, may help improve GERD symptoms by promoting better sleep and reducing inflammation in the esophagus.

By making these dietary changes and adopting healthy lifestyle habits, you can effectively manage acid reflux and improve your digestive health. However, if symptoms persist despite dietary modifications, it's essential to consult with a healthcare professional for further evaluation and treatment.

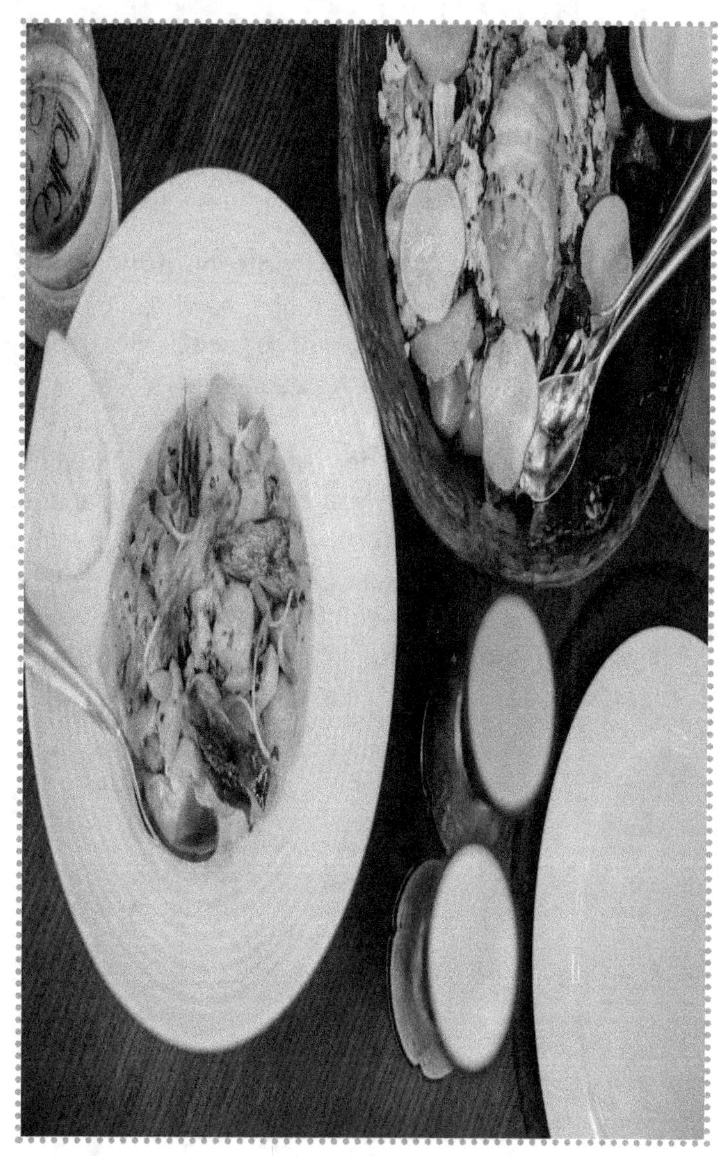

# CHAPTER TWO

## 2.  Fundamentals of an Acid Reflux Diet

Acid reflux, sometimes referred to as gastroesophageal reflux disease (GERD), is an irritable and uncomfortable condition that happens when stomach acid backs up into the esophagus. Managing acid reflux often involves dietary changes to minimize symptoms and promote better digestion. Here are the key fundamentals of an acid reflux diet:

1. **Portion Control:** Eating large meals can put pressure on the stomach and increase the likelihood of acid reflux. Instead, opt for smaller, more frequent meals throughout the day to prevent overeating and reduce stomach pressure.

2. **Meal Timing:** It's essential to allow enough time for digestion before lying down or going to bed. Aim to eat meals at least two to three hours before lying down to give your body enough time to digest food properly.

3. **Stay Upright:** After eating, remain upright for at least 30 minutes to allow gravity to help keep stomach acid down. Avoid lying down immediately after meals to prevent acid reflux symptoms.

4. **Hydration:** Drinking plenty of water throughout the day can help dilute stomach acid and promote better digestion. However, it's best to avoid drinking large amounts of fluids with meals, as this can contribute to acid reflux.

5. **Healthy Eating Habits:** Choose a balanced diet rich in fruits, vegetables, lean proteins, and whole grains. Avoiding processed foods, high-fat meals, and spicy foods can help reduce the risk of acid reflux episodes.

## 2.1   Basic Principles of an Acid Reflux Diet

An acid reflux diet focuses on minimizing foods and beverages that can trigger symptoms while incorporating options that promote better digestion and reduce irritation. Here are the basic principles to follow:

1. **Low-Acid Foods:** Acidic foods and beverages can exacerbate acid reflux symptoms. Opt for low-acid options such as bananas, melons, oatmeal, and whole-grain bread instead of citrus fruits, tomatoes, and vinegar.

2. **Lean Proteins:** Choose lean protein sources such as poultry, fish, tofu, and legumes instead of high-fat meats like bacon, sausage, and

fried chicken. Acid reflux is less common and easier to digest with lean proteins.

3. **Complex Carbohydrates:** Focus on complex carbohydrates such as whole grains, brown rice, quinoa, and sweet potatoes. These foods provide essential nutrients and fiber while being gentle on the digestive system.

4. **Healthy Fats:** Incorporate sources of healthy fats such as avocado, nuts, seeds, and olive oil into your diet. Avoid saturated and trans fats found in fried foods, processed snacks, and fatty meats, as they can worsen acid reflux symptoms.

5. **Limit Trigger Foods:** Identify and limit foods and beverages that commonly trigger acid reflux, such as spicy foods, chocolate, caffeine, carbonated drinks, and alcohol. Keeping a food diary can help pinpoint specific triggers and avoid them accordingly.

## 2.2 Foods to Avoid to Minimize Acid Reflux Symptoms

Certain foods and beverages are known to trigger or exacerbate acid reflux symptoms. By avoiding these items, you can minimize discomfort and reduce the frequency of acid reflux episodes. These foods should be avoided:

1. **Citrus Fruits:** Oranges, grapefruits, lemons, and limes are highly acidic and can irritate the esophagus, leading to acid reflux symptoms.

2. **Tomatoes:** Tomatoes and tomato-based products, such as pasta sauce and ketchup, are acidic and can trigger heartburn and reflux.

3. **Spicy Foods:** Peppers, chili peppers, hot sauces, and spicy seasonings can irritate the esophagus and exacerbate acid reflux symptoms.

4. **Chocolate:** Chocolate contains methylxanthine, which relaxes the lower esophageal sphincter (LES) and allows stomach acid to reflux into the esophagus.

5. **Caffeine:** Coffee, tea, soda, and energy drinks contain caffeine, which can relax the LES and increase the risk of acid reflux.

6. **Carbonated Drinks:** Carbonated beverages, including soda and sparkling water, can distend the stomach and increase pressure, leading to acid reflux symptoms.

7. **Fatty Foods:** High-fat meals, fried foods, fatty cuts of meat, and full-fat dairy products can delay stomach emptying and contribute to acid reflux.

8. **Alcohol**:** Alcohol relaxes the LES and can increase stomach acid production, making it more likely for acid to reflux into the esophagus.

## 2.3    Recommended Foods for Acid Reflux Relief

While some foods can exacerbate acid reflux symptoms, others can provide relief and support digestive health. Incorporating these foods into your diet may help alleviate discomfort and reduce the frequency of reflux episodes. Here are some recommended options:

1. **Non-Citrus Fruits:** Choose fruits such as bananas, apples, pears, and melons, which are low in acid and less likely to trigger reflux.

2. **Vegetables:** Opt for non-acidic vegetables like broccoli, carrots, green beans, and leafy greens, which are rich in vitamins, minerals, and fiber.

3. **Oatmeal:** Oatmeal is a nutritious and filling breakfast option that can help absorb stomach acid and provide long-lasting energy.

4. **Ginger:** Ginger has natural anti-inflammatory properties and can help soothe the digestive tract.

Enjoy ginger tea or incorporate fresh ginger into your meals for added relief.

5. **Lean Proteins:** Choose lean sources of protein such as chicken, turkey, fish, and tofu, which are easier to digest and less likely to trigger acid reflux.

6. **Whole Grains:** Opt for whole grains such as brown rice, quinoa, barley, and whole-grain bread, which provide fiber and essential nutrients without causing irritation.

7. **Healthy Fats:** Incorporate sources of healthy fats like avocado, nuts, seeds, and olive oil into your meals to support digestive health and reduce inflammation.

8. **Non-Caffeinated Beverages:** Drink plenty of water, herbal teas, and non-citrus juices to stay hydrated without exacerbating acid reflux symptoms.

By following these guidelines and making mindful dietary choices, you can better manage acid reflux symptoms and improve overall digestive health. Always pay attention to what your body tells you, and modify your diet to suit your needs.

# CHAPTER THREE

## Key Components of an Acid Reflux Diet:

When it comes to managing acid reflux, your diet plays a crucial role. Certain foods can trigger symptoms like heartburn, regurgitation, and chest pain, while others can soothe and alleviate discomfort. Here are some key components of an acid reflux diet:

1. **Low-Acid Foods:** Opt for foods that are less acidic to minimize irritation to the esophagus. This includes fruits like bananas, melons, and apples, as well as vegetables like carrots, peas, and broccoli.

2. **Lean Proteins:** Choose lean sources of protein such as poultry, fish, and tofu. These options are easier to digest and less likely to cause reflux symptoms compared to fatty cuts of meat.

3. **Complex Carbohydrates:** Incorporate whole grains like brown rice, quinoa, and oats into your meals. These complex carbohydrates provide sustained energy without triggering acid reflux.

4. **Healthy Fats:** Include sources of healthy fats such as avocados, nuts, and seeds in

moderation. These fats can help keep you feeling satisfied without exacerbating reflux symptoms.

5. **Non-Citrus Fruits:** While citrus fruits are acidic and can worsen reflux, non-citrus options like berries, pears, and grapes are generally well-tolerated and provide important nutrients and antioxidants.

6. **Non-Carbonated Beverages:** Stick to water, herbal teas, and diluted fruit juices instead of carbonated drinks, which can contribute to bloating and reflux symptoms.

7. **Low-Fat Dairy:** Opt for low-fat or fat-free dairy products like milk, yogurt, and cheese. These can be beneficial for some people with acid reflux, but be mindful of individual tolerance levels.

8. **Herbs and Spices:** Use herbs and spices like ginger, turmeric, and cinnamon to flavor your meals instead of relying on acidic or spicy seasonings that can trigger reflux.

## Dietary Modifications to Reduce Acid Reflux Symptoms:

In addition to focusing on the right foods, there are several dietary modifications you can make to help reduce acid reflux symptoms:

1. **Smaller, More Frequent Meals:** Instead of eating large meals, try eating smaller portions more frequently throughout the day. This can help prevent overeating, which can contribute to reflux.

2. **Avoid Trigger Foods:** Identify and avoid foods that trigger your acid reflux symptoms. Common triggers include spicy foods, citrus fruits, tomatoes, onions, garlic, chocolate, caffeine, and alcohol.

3. **Limit Acidic and Spicy Foods:** While some acidic and spicy foods can be tolerated in moderation, it's important to limit your intake, especially if they tend to exacerbate your reflux symptoms.

4. **Stay Upright After Eating:** Avoid lying down or reclining immediately after eating, as this can increase the risk of acid reflux. Instead, remain upright for at least two to three hours after meals.

5. **Don't Eat Before Bed:** Aim to finish eating at least two to three hours before bedtime to give

your stomach time to digest food before lying down. This can help prevent nighttime reflux symptoms.

6. **Elevate the Head of Your Bed:** If you experience nighttime reflux, try elevating the head of your bed by placing blocks or risers under the legs. Stomach acid can be kept from flowing back into the esophagus by this small incline.

7. **Chew Gum:** Chewing sugar-free gum after meals can stimulate saliva production, which can help neutralize stomach acid and reduce reflux symptoms.

## Importance of Portion Control and Meal Timing:

Portion control and meal timing are crucial aspects of managing acid reflux:

1. **Prevents Overeating:** Eating large meals can put pressure on the lower esophageal sphincter (LES), the muscle that controls the opening between the esophagus and the stomach. When the LES is weakened or relaxed, stomach acid can flow back into the esophagus, leading to reflux symptoms. By controlling portion sizes, you can reduce the risk of overeating and minimize pressure on the LES.

2. **Reduces Pressure on the Stomach:**
Eating smaller, more frequent meals throughout the day can help prevent excessive distention of the stomach, which can contribute to acid reflux. Large meals can cause the stomach to expand, putting pressure on the LES and increasing the likelihood of reflux.

3. **Promotes Proper Digestion:** Eating at regular intervals and avoiding large meals before bedtime allows your body to digest food more efficiently. When you give your stomach an adequate amount of time to process food before lying down, you can help prevent reflux symptoms that occur when stomach contents flow back into the esophagus.

4. **Enhances Nutrient Absorption:** Portion control and meal timing can also improve nutrient absorption by allowing your body to effectively break down and absorb nutrients from food. This can contribute to overall digestive health and may help alleviate symptoms of acid reflux.

5. **Supports Weight Management:** Controlling portion sizes and eating at regular intervals can support weight management efforts, which is important for reducing the risk of acid reflux. Excess weight, especially around the abdomen, can put pressure on the stomach and LES, leading to reflux symptoms.

6. **Promotes Better Sleep:** Eating smaller meals and avoiding heavy, rich foods before bedtime can help prevent nighttime reflux symptoms, allowing you to sleep more comfortably and wake up feeling refreshed.

## Balancing Macronutrients for Digestive Health:

Achieving a balance of macronutrients—carbohydrates, proteins, and fats—is essential for promoting digestive health and managing acid reflux:

1. **Carbohydrates:** Choose complex carbohydrates like whole grains, fruits, and vegetables, which provide fiber and essential nutrients while promoting digestive regularity. Avoid refined carbohydrates and sugary foods, which can contribute to bloating and discomfort.

2. **Proteins:** Opt for lean sources of protein such as poultry, fish, tofu, beans, and legumes, which are easier to digest and less likely to trigger reflux symptoms compared to fatty cuts of meat. Protein is important for repairing tissues and supporting overall health.

3. **Fats:** Include healthy fats like avocados, nuts, seeds, and olive oil in moderation, as they play a role in nutrient absorption and satiety. Avoid excessive consumption of saturated and trans fats, which can contribute to inflammation and digestive issues.

4. **Fiber:** Ensure an adequate intake of dietary fiber from fruits, vegetables, whole grains, and legumes to support digestive health and prevent constipation. Fiber helps promote regular bowel movements and may reduce the risk of reflux by preventing food from lingering in the stomach.

5. **Hydration:** Drink plenty of water throughout the day to stay hydrated and support optimal digestion. Adequate hydration helps keep stool soft and facilitates the movement of food through the digestive tract, reducing the risk of reflux and other gastrointestinal issues.

6. **Meal Composition:** Aim to create balanced meals that include a combination of carbohydrates, proteins, and fats to promote satiety and stabilize blood sugar levels. Experiment with different meal combinations to find what works best for you and helps minimize reflux symptoms.

By focusing on these dietary principles—choosing the right foods, making dietary modifications, practicing portion control and meal timing, and balancing macronutrients—you can effectively manage acid reflux and promote digestive health. Remember to listen to your body and work with your healthcare provider to develop a personalized approach that meets your individual needs and preferences.

# CHAPTER FOUR

## 4. Understanding Trigger Foods under acid reflux

Truly, acid reflux can be quite painful! It's that burning sensation you get in your chest when stomach acid creeps up into your esophagus. While it can be caused by various factors like lifestyle habits and medical conditions, what you eat plays a big role in triggering it. These trigger foods can vary from person to person, but there are some common culprits that tend to aggravate acid reflux for many people.

## 4.1 Identifying Personal Trigger Foods

When it comes to managing acid reflux, figuring out your personal trigger foods is key. These are the foods that seem to set off your symptoms or make them worse. Keeping a food diary can be super helpful in identifying them. Jot down everything you consume, including drinks, and any after-effects symptoms you may feel. Over time, you may start to notice patterns and can pinpoint which foods are causing trouble for you.

## 4.2   Common Foods That Aggravate Acid Reflux

Now, let's talk about some common foods that tend to aggravate acid reflux for a lot of folks. One big culprit is spicy foods. They can irritate the lining of your esophagus and make that burning sensation even worse. Fatty foods are another no-no. They can relax the muscle that controls the opening between your esophagus and stomach, allowing acid to sneak up more easily. And let's not forget about citrus fruits and juices. While they're packed with vitamin C, they're also highly acidic, which can spell trouble for those with acid reflux.

## 4.3   Strategies for Avoiding Trigger Foods

So, how can you avoid these trigger foods and keep your acid reflux in check? First off, try to steer clear of spicy and fatty foods as much as possible. Opt for milder options instead. When it comes to citrus fruits, you don't have to cut them out completely, but it's a good idea to enjoy them in moderation. And don't forget about portion control. Eating smaller meals throughout the day can help prevent overeating, which can exacerbate acid reflux symptoms.

Another strategy is to pay attention to how you eat. Eating too quickly or lying down right after a meal can increase the likelihood of acid reflux. Instead, try to eat slowly and chew your food thoroughly. And be sure to stay upright for at least a couple of hours after eating to give your stomach time to digest properly.

In addition to watching what you eat, paying attention to when you eat can also make a difference. Avoid eating large meals or heavy snacks right before bedtime, as lying down can make it easier for acid to creep up into your esophagus. Instead, aim to eat your last meal of the day at least a few hours before hitting the hay.

Lastly, don't forget about lifestyle factors that can contribute to acid reflux. Things like smoking, excessive alcohol consumption, and being overweight can all increase your risk. So, if you're a smoker, consider kicking the habit. And if you enjoy a drink now and then, try to keep it to a minimum. Maintaining a healthy weight through diet and exercise can also help reduce your symptoms.

Finally, managing acid reflux involves a combination of identifying your personal trigger foods and making lifestyle changes to avoid them. By paying attention to what you eat, how you eat, and when you eat, you can help keep those pesky symptoms at bay and enjoy better digestive health overall.

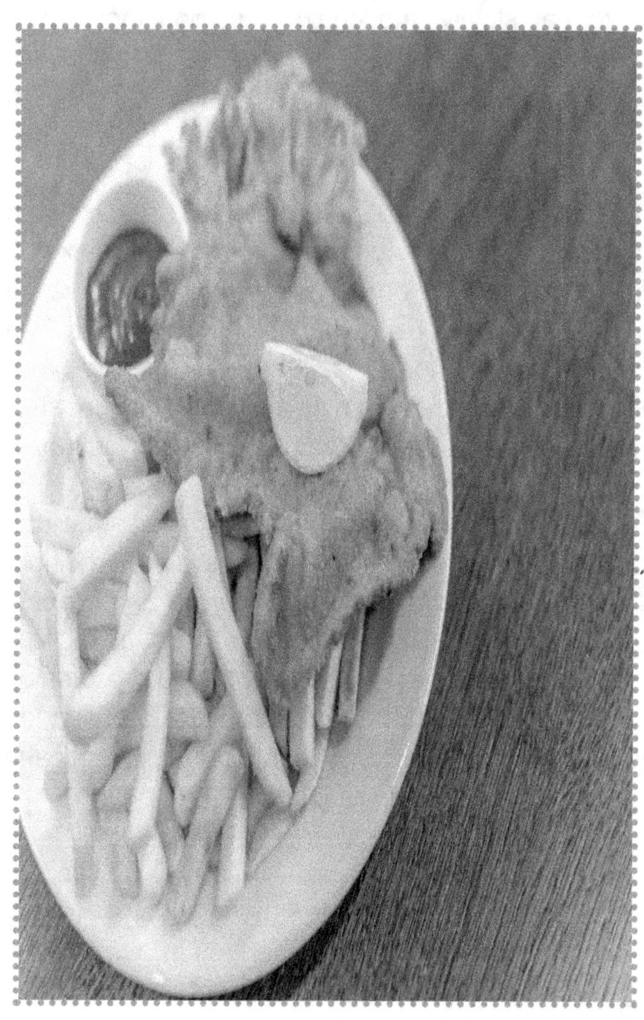

# CHAPTER FIVE

## 5.  Lifestyle Changes for Acid Reflux Management:

Acid reflux, also known as gastroesophageal reflux disease (GERD), can be a real discomfort in your daily life. But fear not, there are several lifestyle changes you can make to manage and alleviate the symptoms.

### 1. **Dietary Adjustments:**

- Monitor your food intake and identify trigger foods that worsen your symptoms. Common culprits include spicy foods, citrus fruits, tomatoes, chocolate, caffeine, and fatty or fried foods.

- Opt for smaller, more frequent meals rather than large meals, which can put pressure on the stomach and increase the likellhood of acid reflux.

- Eat slowly and chew your food thoroughly to aid digestion and reduce the risk of reflux.

2. **Maintain a Healthy Weight:**

- Excess weight, especially around the abdomen, can put pressure on the stomach and lead to acid reflux. Even a tiny weight loss can have a big impact on symptoms.

- Incorporate regular exercise into your routine to help with weight management and improve overall digestive health.

3. **Modify Sleeping Habits:**

- Elevate the head of your bed by 6 to 8 inches to prevent stomach acid from flowing back into the esophagus while you sleep.

- Avoid eating large meals or snacks close to bedtime, as lying down shortly after eating can trigger or worsen symptoms of acid reflux.

4. **Quit Smoking:**

- Smoking weakens the lower esophageal sphincter (LES), the muscle that helps prevent stomach acid from flowing back into the esophagus. Quitting smoking can significantly reduce the frequency and severity of acid reflux symptoms.

5. **Limit Alcohol Consumption:**

   - Alcohol can relax the LES and irritate the lining of the esophagus, leading to increased acid reflux symptoms. Limiting your alcohol intake, especially before bedtime, can help alleviate symptoms.

6. **Stress Management:**

   - Stress and anxiety can exacerbate acid reflux symptoms by increasing stomach acid production and disrupting digestion. Incorporate stress-reducing techniques into your daily routine, such as mindfulness meditation, deep breathing exercises, yoga, or engaging in hobbies you enjoy.


# 5.1 Importance of Weight Management in Acid Reflux:

Maintaining a healthy weight is crucial for managing acid reflux and reducing the frequency and severity of symptoms. Here's why weight management plays such a significant role:

1. **Reduces Pressure on the Stomach:**

   - Excess weight, particularly around the abdomen, puts increased pressure on the stomach and can cause the contents to reflux back into the esophagus. By shedding excess pounds, you can alleviate this pressure and reduce the likelihood of acid reflux episodes.

2. **Improves Esophageal Function:**

   - Carrying excess weight can weaken the lower esophageal sphincter (LES), the muscle that acts as a barrier between the stomach and the esophagus. When the LES is weakened, stomach acid is more likely to flow back into the esophagus, causing symptoms of acid reflux. Losing weight can help strengthen the LES and improve its function.

3. **Decreases Acid Production:**

   - Adipose tissue, or fat cells, produce hormones and chemicals that can increase stomach acid production, exacerbating acid reflux symptoms. By reducing overall body fat through weight management, you can lower the levels of these substances and decrease acid production.

4. **Enhances Overall Digestive Health:**

- Maintaining a healthy weight through proper diet and exercise promotes overall digestive health. Eating a balanced diet and engaging in regular physical activity can improve digestion, reduce bloating and gas, and minimize the occurrence of acid reflux episodes.

In summary, weight management is essential for managing acid reflux because it reduces pressure on the stomach, improves esophageal function, decreases acid production, and enhances overall digestive health. By achieving and maintaining a healthy weight, you can effectively alleviate symptoms and improve your quality of life.

## 5.2   Impact of Smoking and Alcohol on Acid Reflux:

Smoking and alcohol consumption can have detrimental effects on acid reflux, exacerbating symptoms and increasing the risk of complications. Here's how smoking and alcohol impact acid reflux:

1.    **Smoking    Weakens    the    Lower Esophageal Sphincter (LES):**

   - The chemicals in cigarettes can weaken the LES, the muscle that acts as a barrier between the stomach and the esophagus. When the LES is weakened, stomach acid is more likely to flow back into the esophagus, causing symptoms of acid reflux such as heartburn, regurgitation, and chest pain.

## 2. **Increases Acid Production:**

   - Smoking stimulates the production of stomach acid, further contributing to acid reflux symptoms. The increased acidity in the stomach can exacerbate irritation of the esophagus and worsen symptoms.

## 3. **Delays Esophageal Healing:**

   - Smoking impairs the body's ability to heal damaged tissues, including the lining of the esophagus. Continued smoking can prolong the healing process and increase the risk of complications such as esophageal ulcers, strictures, or Barrett's esophagus.

## 4. **Alcohol Relaxes the Lower Esophageal Sphincter (LES):**

- Alcohol consumption can relax the LES, making it easier for stomach acid to reflux into the esophagus. This can lead to symptoms of acid reflux and increase the risk of complications.

## 5. **Irritates the Esophageal Lining:**

- Alcohol is a known irritant to the lining of the esophagus. Excessive alcohol consumption can cause inflammation and damage to the esophageal mucosa, exacerbating symptoms of acid reflux and increasing the risk of complications such as esophagitis or esophageal bleeding.

## 6. **Triggers Acid Reflux Symptoms:**

- Both smoking and alcohol consumption are known triggers for acid reflux symptoms. Individuals with GERD are advised to avoid or limit their intake of tobacco and alcohol to reduce the frequency and severity of symptoms.

Lastly,, smoking and alcohol consumption can significantly worsen acid reflux symptoms by weakening the LES, increasing stomach acid production, delaying esophageal healing, and irritating the esophageal lining. Minimizing or eliminating smoking and alcohol intake is essential for effectively managing acid reflux and reducing the risk of complications.

## 5.3 Stress Management Techniques for Acid Reflux Relief:

Stress is a common trigger for acid reflux symptoms and can exacerbate the condition. Incorporating stress management techniques into your daily routine can help alleviate symptoms and improve your overall quality of life. Here are some effective stress management techniques for acid reflux relief:

### 1. **Mindfulness Meditation:**

- Mindfulness meditation entails paying attention to the here and now while letting go of judgment. Practicing mindfulness meditation regularly can help reduce stress and anxiety, which are known triggers for acid reflux symptoms.

### 2. **Deep Breathing Exercises:**

- Deep breathing exercises, such as diaphragmatic breathing or belly breathing, can activate the body's relaxation response and reduce stress levels. Practice deep breathing for a few minutes each day or during times of increased stress to promote relaxation and alleviate acid reflux symptoms.

### 3. **Progressive Muscle Relaxation (PMR):**

- PMR involves systematically tensing and relaxing different muscle groups in the body to promote relaxation and reduce tension. Practicing PMR regularly can help reduce muscle tension, relieve stress, and alleviate symptoms of acid reflux.

### 4. **Yoga:**

- Yoga combines physical postures, breathing exercises, and meditation to promote relaxation, reduce stress,

and improve overall well-being. Certain yoga poses, such as gentle twists and forward bends, can also aid digestion and alleviate symptoms of acid reflux.

### 5. **Regular Exercise:**

- Engaging in regular physical activity, such as walking, swimming, or cycling, can help reduce stress levels and promote relaxation. Aim for at least 30 minutes of moderate exercise most days of the week to improve your mood and alleviate acid reflux symptoms.

6. **Healthy Lifestyle Habits:**

- In addition to specific stress management techniques, adopting healthy lifestyle habits can also help reduce stress and improve overall well-being. Get an adequate amount of sleep each night, maintain a balanced diet, stay hydrated, and avoid excessive caffeine and alcohol intake.

By incorporating stress management techniques into your daily routine, you can effectively reduce stress levels, alleviate symptoms of acid reflux, and improve your overall quality of life. Experiment with different techniques to find what works best for you, and make stress management a priority in your acid reflux management plan.

# CHAPTER SIX

## 6.      Meal Planning and Preparation

Meal planning and preparation are essential aspects of maintaining a healthy diet, especially for those managing acid reflux. Planning ahead can help you choose foods that are less likely to trigger symptoms while ensuring you have nutritious and satisfying meals throughout the week.

Make a weekly meal plan that consists of a range of foods from all the food groups to start. Balance your intake of whole grains, fruits, vegetables, lean proteins, and healthy fats. When planning your meals, consider your personal triggers for acid reflux and try to avoid or limit them.

Once you have your meal plan, it's time to prepare your ingredients. Wash and chop fruits and vegetables, portion out proteins, and pre-cook grains or legumes if needed. Having these items ready to go will make mealtime a breeze, especially on busy days when you're short on time.

Invest in some quality storage containers to help keep your prepped ingredients fresh throughout the week. Mason jars are great for salads and overnight oats, while glass or plastic containers with tight-fitting lids are perfect for storing cooked proteins and chopped vegetables.

## 6.1    Creating Acid Reflux-Friendly Meal Plans

When creating acid reflux-friendly meal plans, it's important to focus on foods that are less likely to trigger symptoms. While everyone's triggers may vary, there are some general guidelines to keep in mind.

Opt for lean proteins such as chicken, turkey, fish, and tofu, which are easier to digest than fatty or fried meats. Incorporate plenty of fruits and vegetables, but be mindful of acidic options like citrus fruits and tomatoes, which can aggravate acid reflux in some people.

Choose whole grains like brown rice, quinoa, and oats over refined grains like white rice and bread. These high-fiber options can help keep you feeling full and satisfied while also supporting digestive health.

Limit or avoid spicy foods, caffeine, alcohol, and carbonated beverages, as these can all exacerbate acid reflux symptoms. Instead, flavor your meals with herbs, spices, and seasonings that are less likely to irritate your stomach, such as ginger, turmeric, and parsley.

## 6.2   Tips for Cooking and Seasoning Without Aggravating Acid Reflux

Cooking and seasoning without aggravating acid reflux may require some adjustments, but it's entirely possible to create delicious meals that won't leave you feeling uncomfortable. Here are some tips to help you cook and season with ease:

1. **Choose cooking methods wisely:** Opt for baking, grilling, steaming, or sautéing instead of frying, which can add unnecessary fat and increase the likelihood of triggering reflux.

2. **Use less oil:** While healthy fats are an important part of any diet, too much oil can exacerbate acid reflux symptoms. Try using cooking sprays or non-stick pans to reduce the amount of oil needed in your recipes.

3. **Experiment with herbs and spices:** Get creative with your seasonings by using herbs and spices that add flavor without the acidity. Basil, thyme, oregano, and rosemary are all excellent options to try.

4. **Opt for low-acid ingredients:** When possible, choose low-acid versions of ingredients

like vinegar (such as apple cider vinegar), tomatoes (such as yellow or orange varieties), and citrus fruits (like melons or bananas).

5. **Be mindful of portion sizes:** Eating large meals can put pressure on your stomach and increase the risk of acid reflux. Aim for smaller, more frequent meals throughout the day to help prevent symptoms.

6. **Stay hydrated:** Drinking plenty of water throughout the day can help dilute stomach acid and reduce the risk of reflux. Avoid drinking large amounts of liquid with meals, as this can distend the stomach and increase pressure on the esophageal sphincter.

7. **Listen to your body:** Pay attention to how different foods and cooking methods affect your symptoms, and make adjustments as needed. Everyone's triggers are unique, so it's important to find what works best for you.

## 6.3  Meal Prepping for Busy Lifestyles

Meal prepping is a lifesaver for busy individuals looking to maintain a healthy diet while juggling a hectic schedule. By preparing meals in advance, you can save time, reduce stress, and ensure you always have nutritious options on hand.

Start by carving out some time each week to plan your meals and prep your ingredients. Choose recipes that are simple, versatile, and easy to batch cook, such as soups, stews, stir-fries, and casseroles.

Invest in quality storage containers that are both microwave and freezer-safe, so you can easily reheat and enjoy your prepped meals throughout the week. Divide larger dishes into individual portions for quick grab-and-go lunches or dinners.

Get creative with your meal prep by mixing and matching ingredients to create different flavor combinations. For example, roast a variety of vegetables at the beginning of the week and use them in salads, wraps, and grain bowls.

Don't forget about snacks! Prep healthy snacks like cut-up fruits and vegetables, hummus and whole-grain crackers, or Greek yogurt with granola to keep you satisfied between meals.

Finally, embrace the freezer! Many meals can be prepped ahead of time and stored in the freezer for later use. Soups, chili, casseroles, and even cooked grains and proteins can all be frozen and reheated with ease.

By incorporating meal planning, acid reflux-friendly recipes, mindful cooking techniques, and efficient meal prepping into your routine, you can enjoy delicious and nutritious meals without aggravating your symptoms, even with a busy lifestyle.

# CHAPTER SEVEN

## 7.   Soothing Beverages for Acid Reflux Relief: [Your Guide to Hydration and Comfort]

Dealing with acid reflux can be a real pain, quite literally. It's that uncomfortable feeling in your chest, the regurgitation of sour-tasting liquid, and the constant worry about what you can and cannot drink. But fear not! With the right knowledge and choices, you can find relief and enjoy a variety of beverages without aggravating your symptoms. In this guide, we'll explore beverages tailored to provide relief for acid reflux, tips for staying hydrated, and how to navigate the tricky terrain of coffee, tea, and carbonated drinks.

### 7.1  Beverages for Acid Reflux Relief:

When it comes to soothing acid reflux symptoms, not all beverages are created equal. Here are some options that can help alleviate discomfort:

1. **Water**: Let's start with the most basic and essential drink – water. Pure, plain water can help dilute stomach acid and wash it back down into the stomach where it belongs. Sip on water throughout the day to stay hydrated and keep acid reflux at bay.

2. **Herbal Tea**: Certain herbal teas have properties that can soothe the digestive tract and reduce acid reflux symptoms. Chamomile tea, in particular, is known for its calming effects on the stomach. Ginger tea is another excellent choice, as ginger can help alleviate nausea and promote digestion.

3. **Aloe Vera Juice**: Aloe vera is not just for soothing sunburns; it can also provide relief for acid reflux. Aloe vera juice can help reduce inflammation in the esophagus and soothe irritation caused by acid reflux.

4. **Almond Milk**: If you're looking for a dairy alternative that won't exacerbate acid reflux, almond milk is a great option. It's alkaline nature can help neutralize stomach acid and provide relief from heartburn.

5. **Coconut Water**: Coconut water is not only refreshing but also naturally alkaline. It can help neutralize stomach acid and provide hydration without aggravating acid reflux symptoms.

## 7.2  Hydration and Acid Reflux:

Staying hydrated is crucial for overall health, but for acid reflux sufferers, it's especially important to choose beverages wisely. Here are some tips for staying hydrated without worsening your symptoms:

1. **Sip Throughout the Day**: Instead of chugging large amounts of liquid at once, sip on beverages slowly throughout the day. This can help prevent your stomach from becoming too full, which can exacerbate acid reflux.

2. **Avoid Trigger Beverages**: Certain beverages, such as citrus juices, caffeinated drinks, and carbonated beverages, can trigger acid reflux symptoms. Opt for non-acidic, non-caffeinated options to stay hydrated without causing discomfort.

3. **Monitor Your Intake**: Pay attention to how your body responds to different beverages. If you notice that a particular drink consistently triggers acid reflux symptoms, consider cutting it out of your diet or consuming it in moderation.

4. **Choose Low-Acid Options**: When selecting beverages, opt for low-acid options whenever possible. This includes drinks like herbal teas, alkaline water, and non-citrus juices.

## 7.3   Best Beverage Choices for Acid Reflux Sufferers:

So, what are the best beverage choices for acid reflux sufferers? Here's a handy list to keep in mind:

1. **Water**: Plain, simple water is always a safe bet for staying hydrated and soothing acid reflux symptoms.

2. **Herbal Teas**: Chamomile, ginger, and licorice root teas are all excellent choices for calming the digestive tract and reducing acid reflux.

3. **Aloe Vera Juice**: This soothing juice can help reduce inflammation and provide relief from acid reflux discomfort.

4. **Almond Milk**: A dairy-free alternative that's gentle on the stomach and can help neutralize acid.

5. **Coconut Water**: Naturally alkaline and hydrating, coconut water is a refreshing option for acid reflux sufferers.

## 7.4    Planning of Coffee, Tea, and Carbonated Drinks:

Coffee, tea, and carbonated drinks are popular beverages enjoyed by many, but they can be problematic for acid reflux sufferers. Here's how to navigate them:

1. **Coffee**: Coffee is highly acidic and can trigger acid reflux symptoms in some people. If you can't bear to part with your morning cup of joe, try switching to a low-acid coffee blend or opting for decaffeinated coffee.

2. **Tea**: While herbal teas are generally safe for acid reflux sufferers, black and green teas contain caffeine, which can exacerbate symptoms. If you enjoy tea, opt for herbal varieties or decaffeinated options.

3. **Carbonated Drinks**: The bubbles in carbonated drinks can expand in your stomach, causing pressure and increasing the likelihood of acid reflux. It's best to avoid carbonated beverages altogether or opt for flat versions.

Lastly,
Finding relief from acid reflux doesn't mean giving up on enjoying beverages altogether. By making mindful choices and opting for soothing options,

you can stay hydrated and comfortable without exacerbating your symptoms. Remember to listen to your body and pay attention to how different drinks affect you. With a little trial and error, you can find the perfect beverages to keep acid reflux at bay while quenching your thirst. Cheers to good health!

# CHAPTER EIGHT

## 8.    Helming to Snacking and Desserts with Acid Reflux: [Your Comprehensive Guide]

Dealing with acid reflux can put a damper on your snacking and dessert options, but it doesn't have to mean saying goodbye to all your favorite treats. With a bit of know-how and creativity, you can still enjoy delicious snacks and desserts without triggering discomfort. In this guide, we'll explore acid reflux-friendly snack ideas, dessert options that won't cause issues, and the importance of portion control and timing when it comes to snacking.

## 8.1    Acid Reflux-Friendly Snack Ideas:

When it comes to snacking with acid reflux, choosing the right foods is key. Opt for snacks that are low in fat and acidity, as these are less likely to trigger symptoms. Here are some acid reflux-friendly snack ideas to consider:

1. **Oatmeal with Banana:** Oatmeal is gentle on the stomach and can help absorb excess acid. Top it with sliced banana for added flavor and nutrients.

2. **Greek Yogurt with Honey:** Greek yogurt is rich in protein and probiotics, which can promote digestive health. Add a drizzle of honey for sweetness without the acidity of other sweeteners.

3. **Rice Cakes with Almond Butter:** Rice cakes are a bland option that won't irritate the esophagus. Spread them with almond butter for a satisfying snack that's easy on the stomach.

4. **Vegetable Sticks with Hummus:** Crunchy vegetables like carrots, cucumber, and bell peppers are low in acidity and high in fiber. Pair them with a creamy, non-acidic hummus for a nutritious snack.

5. **Baked Apples:** Apples are typically off-limits for acid reflux sufferers, but baking them can make them easier to digest. Sprinkle with cinnamon for added flavor.

## 8.2    Dessert Options That Won't Trigger Acid Reflux:

When it comes to dessert, it's all about moderation and choosing options that are less likely to cause discomfort. Here are some dessert options that are less likely to trigger acid reflux:

1. **Angel Food Cake:** Light and fluffy, angel food cake is lower in fat than other types of cake, making it a better option for those with acid reflux. Serve it with some fresh berries for a taste boost.

2. **Frozen Yogurt:** Unlike ice cream, frozen yogurt tends to be lower in fat and acidity, making it a safer choice for dessert. Just be mindful of portion sizes and avoid toppings that could trigger symptoms.

3. **Banana "Nice" Cream:** Blend frozen bananas until creamy for a dairy-free, naturally sweet dessert option. You can add cocoa powder or peanut butter for extra flavor without the acidity.

4. **Ginger Cookies:** Ginger is known for its digestive properties and can help alleviate nausea and indigestion. Bake up a batch of ginger cookies using whole wheat flour and natural sweeteners like honey or maple syrup.

5. **Rice Pudding:** Creamy and soothing, rice pudding is gentle on the stomach and less likely to cause discomfort. Opt for a recipe made with almond milk for a dairy-free option.

## 8.3    Portion Control and Timing for Snacking:

In addition to choosing the right foods, it's important to practice portion control and mindful snacking to prevent acid reflux symptoms. Here are some tips for snacking with acid reflux:

1. **Stick to Small Portions:** Instead of mindlessly munching on large quantities of snacks, portion out small servings to prevent overeating and reduce the risk of triggering symptoms.

2. **Avoid Late-Night Snacking:** Eating close to bedtime can increase the likelihood of acid reflux symptoms, so try to avoid late-night snacking whenever possible. If you do need a snack before bed, opt for something light and easy to digest.

3. **Space Out Snacks:** Instead of grazing throughout the day, try to space out your snacks to give your digestive system time to process food properly. Aim for snacks that are at least two to three hours apart from your main meals.

4. **Listen to Your Body:** Pay attention to how your body reacts to different foods and adjust your snacking habits accordingly. If you notice that certain snacks consistently trigger symptoms, it may be best to avoid them altogether.

Lastly,
Living with acid reflux doesn't mean sacrificing flavor and enjoyment when it comes to snacks and desserts. By choosing the right foods, practicing portion control, and being mindful of timing, you can still indulge in delicious treats without discomfort. Experiment with the snack and dessert options provided, and don't be afraid to get creative in the kitchen. With a little planning and moderation, you can snack and satisfy your sweet tooth while keeping acid reflux symptoms at bay.

# CHAPTER NINE

## 9.     Eating Out and Social Situations under Acid Reflux

When you're dealing with acid reflux, eating out and navigating social situations can feel like tiptoeing through a culinary minefield. But fear not, there are strategies to help you enjoy dining out and socializing without triggering painful reflux symptoms.

First off, let's talk about what makes dining out challenging for those with acid reflux. Restaurants often serve dishes loaded with trigger foods like spicy sauces, citrus fruits, fatty meats, and tomatoes - all of which can set off that uncomfortable burning sensation. Plus, the temptation of indulging in rich desserts and alcohol can be hard to resist.

So, what can you do to tackle this gastronomic gauntlet? It starts with being proactive and doing a little research. Before heading out, take a peek at the restaurant's menu online. Look for options that are less likely to cause reflux, such as grilled chicken or fish, steamed veggies, and plain pasta. Many restaurants nowadays even label their menu items as "low acid" or "acid-friendly," making your job easier.

When ordering, don't be afraid to make special requests. Ask for sauces and dressings on the side so you can control the amount, and request grilled or baked preparations instead of fried. Most restaurants are more than happy to accommodate dietary needs, so don't hesitate to speak up.

Another tip is to eat slowly and mindfully. Take your time savoring each bite, and stop eating when you start to feel full. Overeating can put pressure on your stomach, leading to reflux symptoms.

Now, let's move on to social situations. Whether it's a dinner party, barbecue, or cocktail hour, social gatherings often revolve around food and drinks. But that doesn't mean you have to sit on the sidelines while everyone else indulges.

One strategy is to eat a small meal or snack before heading to the event. This can help prevent overeating and reduce the likelihood of reflux symptoms later on. You can also bring your own dish to share, ensuring there's at least one reflux-friendly option available.

When it comes to drinks, stick to water or non-acidic beverages like herbal tea or diluted fruit juice. Avoid carbonated drinks and alcohol, as they can exacerbate reflux symptoms.

Lastly, don't be afraid to excuse yourself from the table if you're feeling uncomfortable. Politely explain to your host that you're dealing with acid reflux and need to take a break. Most people will understand and won't pressure you to keep eating or drinking.

Lastly, dining out and socializing with acid reflux may require a bit of extra planning and effort, but it's entirely possible to enjoy yourself without suffering the consequences. By making smart food choices, advocating for your dietary needs, and being mindful of your body's signals, you can navigate any social situation with ease.

## 9.1　Strategies for Dining Out with Acid Reflux

Dining out with acid reflux can feel like steering a culinary obstacle course, but with the right strategies, you can enjoy a meal without triggering painful symptoms. Here are some tips to help you dine out with confidence:

1. **Do your homework**: Before heading to a restaurant, take a look at the menu online. Look for dishes that are less likely to cause reflux, such as grilled or baked options, lean proteins, and steamed vegetables.

2. **Make special requests**: Don't be afraid to ask for modifications to suit your dietary needs. Request sauces and dressings on the side, opt for grilled instead of fried preparations, and ask about ingredient substitutions.

3. **Eat slowly and mindfully**: Take your time to savor each bite and listen to your body's cues. Stop eating when you start to feel full, as overeating can exacerbate reflux symptoms.

4. **Be prepared**: Consider bringing along antacids or other reflux medications, just in case you need them. Having them on hand can provide peace of mind and help manage symptoms if they arise.

5. **Stay hydrated**: Drink plenty of water throughout your meal to help dilute stomach acid and aid digestion. Avoid carbonated beverages and alcohol, as they can worsen reflux symptoms.

6. **Choose your indulgences wisely**: If you're tempted by dessert or a cocktail, opt for lighter options that are less likely to trigger reflux. Fresh fruit, sorbet, and light cocktails made with non-acidic mixers are good choices.

By following these strategies, you can enjoy dining out without worrying about your acid reflux acting up. Remember to advocate for your dietary needs and listen to your body's signals, and you'll be able to savor your meal with confidence.

## 9.2  Steering Social Gatherings and Events

Social gatherings and events can be challenging to navigate when you have acid reflux, but with a little planning and preparation, you can still enjoy yourself without discomfort. Here are some strategies for steering social gatherings and events:

1. **Plan ahead**: Before attending a social event, find out what food and drinks will be served. If possible, offer to bring a dish that you know is reflux-friendly, ensuring that there's at least one option you can enjoy.

2. **Communicate your needs**: Don't be shy about letting your host know about your dietary restrictions. Explain that you have acid reflux and ask if there will be any options available that won't trigger symptoms.

3. **Be strategic**: Scan the buffet or food spread and identify dishes that are less likely to cause reflux, such as grilled proteins, salads without acidic dressings, and cooked vegetables.

4. **Pace yourself**: Take your time eating and drinking, and be mindful of portion sizes. Avoid overeating, as it can put pressure on your stomach and increase the likelihood of reflux symptoms.

5. **Choose your beverages wisely**: Stick to non-acidic drinks like water, herbal tea, or diluted fruit juice. Avoid carbonated beverages and alcohol, as they can irritate the esophagus and worsen reflux symptoms.

6. **Take breaks**: If you start to feel uncomfortable, don't hesitate to step away from the food and drink. Find a quiet spot to relax and allow your body to settle before returning to the festivities.

By following these strategies, you can navigate social gatherings and events with ease, enjoying the company of others without worrying about your acid reflux flaring up.

## 9.3  Communicating Dietary Needs to Others

Communicating your dietary needs to others can feel daunting, but it's essential for managing your acid reflux and ensuring that you can enjoy meals without discomfort. The following advice can help you explain your dietary requirements to others:

1. **Be upfront**: When dining out or attending social events, don't hesitate to let your host or server know about your dietary restrictions. Explain that you have acid reflux and ask for assistance in finding suitable options.

2. **Offer suggestions**: If possible, provide examples of foods and dishes that you can safely eat. This can help your host or server better understand your needs and make appropriate accommodations.

3. **Be polite but firm**: It's important to advocate for yourself while still being respectful. Firmly communicate your dietary needs, but avoid being confrontational or demanding.

4. **Express gratitude**: Remember to thank your host or server for accommodating your dietary needs. Showing appreciation can help foster positive relationships and encourage future support.

5. **Educate when necessary**: If someone isn't familiar with acid reflux or its dietary implications, take the opportunity to educate them. Explain the symptoms you experience and why certain foods can trigger discomfort.

6. **Be flexible**: While it's important to stick to your dietary restrictions, try to be flexible and open-minded when attending social gatherings. Focus on enjoying the company of others rather than solely on the food.

By effectively communicating your dietary needs to others, you can ensure that your meals are both enjoyable and comfortable, allowing you to fully participate in social events without worrying about acid reflux symptoms.

# CHAPTER TEN

## 10.  Monitoring and Adjusting the Acid Reflux Diet

Ah, acid reflux – that uncomfortable sensation when stomach acid backs up into your esophagus, causing that burning feeling in your chest. If you're dealing with this pesky issue, one of the best ways to manage it is through your diet. But how do you go about monitoring and adjusting your diet to keep those symptoms at bay?

## 10.1  Monitoring Symptoms

First things first, it's crucial to pay attention to your body and the symptoms you experience. Keep a journal where you can jot down when you experience acid reflux symptoms, what you ate prior to them, and any other relevant details. This can help you identify patterns and triggers, making it easier to adjust your diet accordingly.

## 10.2   Keeping Track of Dietary Intake

Next up, let's talk about keeping track of what you eat. This doesn't mean you have to meticulously count every calorie or measure every portion (unless you want to, of course!). Instead, focus on being mindful of what you're putting into your body. Consider using a food diary or a smartphone app to track your meals, snacks, and beverages. Be sure to note any potential trigger foods or drinks that seem to worsen your acid reflux symptoms.

## 10.3   Consulting with Healthcare Professionals

While making dietary changes on your own can be helpful, it's always a good idea to consult with healthcare professionals for guidance. Your doctor or a registered dietitian can provide personalized recommendations based on your specific needs and health history. They can help you identify trigger foods, suggest alternatives, and ensure you're getting all the nutrients your body needs while managing acid reflux.

## 10.4  Making Sustainable Changes

Now, let's talk about making sustainable changes for long-term acid reflux management. It's easy to get caught up in fad diets or drastic restrictions, but these often aren't sustainable in the long run. Rather, concentrate on altering your eating habits gradually and permanently. . Start by gradually reducing or eliminating trigger foods from your diet, while incorporating more foods that are gentle on your digestive system.

## 10.5 Choosing the Right Foods

So, what should you be eating to help manage acid reflux? While everyone's triggers may vary slightly, there are some general guidelines to keep in mind. Opt for lean proteins like chicken, fish, and tofu, as well as plenty of fruits and vegetables. Whole grains, such as oats, brown rice, and quinoa, can also be beneficial. Be sure to drink plenty of water throughout the day to stay hydrated and help prevent acid reflux.

## 10.6 Avoiding Trigger Foods

On the flip side, there are certain foods and drinks that are notorious for triggering acid reflux symptoms. Citrus fruits, tomatoes, chocolate, caffeine, and fizzy drinks are a few examples of these. Keep an eye on how these items affect your symptoms and consider cutting back or eliminating them from your diet if they seem to worsen your acid reflux.

## 10.7 Managing Portion Sizes

In addition to choosing the right foods, paying attention to portion sizes can also play a role in managing acid reflux. Eating large meals can put added pressure on your stomach and increase the likelihood of acid reflux symptoms. Instead, aim for smaller, more frequent meals throughout the day to help keep your digestive system happy and reduce the risk of reflux.

## 10.8 Eating Mindfully

Finally, don't forget the importance of eating mindfully. Eat slowly, give your food a good chewing motion, and pay attention to your body's signals of hunger and fullness. Eating too quickly or mindlessly can lead to overeating, which can exacerbate acid reflux symptoms. By taking the time to savor your meals and listen to your body, you can help prevent discomfort and promote better digestion.

# 10.9     DAILY MEAL PLAN

| S/N | DAILY | MEAL | REMAKE |
| --- | --- | --- | --- |
| 1. | | | |
| | | | |
| | | | |
| | | | |
| | | | |
| | | | |
| | | | |
| | | | |
| | | | |
| | | | |
| | | | |
| | | | |
| | | | |
| | | | |

|  |  |  | 73 |
|---|---|---|---|
|  |  |  |  |
|  |  |  |  |
|  |  |  |  |

|  |  |  |  |
|---|---|---|---|
|  |  |  |  |
|  |  |  |  |
|  |  |  |  |
|  |  |  |  |
|  |  |  |  |
|  |  |  |  |
|  |  |  |  |